Natasha's Joy

Natasha's Joy

The Gift of Life for My Sister

Terri W. Godwin

BJ Publishing
Research Triangle Park, NC

Natasha's Joy:
The Gift of Life for My Sister
By Terri W. Godwin

Lateef Mangum took the photograph
"Mayor Williams Signs Organ Donor Leave Act."
It has been reprinted here with permission.

Library of Congress Control Number: 2007904224

ISBN 13: 978-0-9814761-0-0
ISBN 10: 0-9814761-0-4

Cover and interior design by Peri Poloni-Gabriel

Printed in the United States of America

Books are available at quantity discounts when used for living organ donation awareness campaigns or promotions. For information, please write to: BJ Publishing, Special Markets Department, P.O. Box 12653, Research Triangle Park, NC 27709 or e-mail info@bjpublishingonline.com.

www.bjpublishingonline.com

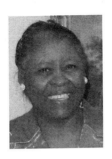

To my mother, Bettie J. Godwin,

whose untimely passing has left an immeasurable void.

Thank you, Mom, for encouraging me

to write this book and share my story with others.

Your vision and foresight are unparalleled.

Contents

Foreword

In 1954, Harvard surgeon Joseph Murray performed the world's first successful kidney transplant, an achievement for which he was awarded the Nobel Prize in Medicine. At that time, there were no therapies available to prevent a recipient from recognizing the new kidney as "foreign" and rejecting it. In fact, the only patients fortunate enough to qualify for transplantation were those with a healthy, identical twin who could serve as the donor, a rare situation indeed. The ensuing decades saw great advances in the ability to manipulate recipients' immune systems such that kidneys are now transplanted routinely across barriers once thought to be insurmountable.

In 2002, the miracle of kidney transplantation was performed 14,779 times in the United States. Although the majority of those kidneys were obtained from deceased donors, 6,240 altruistic individuals made the decision to serve as living donors. One of them was Terri Godwin, who accepted the risks of a major operation to free her sister from the rigors of hemodialysis. To replace the function of kidneys damaged by lupus, Natasha required four-hour sessions on three separate days per week. Although the treatments to rid her system of toxins and excess fluid were lifesaving, the side effects were debilitating. Just as dialysis patients recover from their last session, it is time to go to the next session ... nonstop, every other day, just to survive. It is difficult to work when you are a dialysis patient. It is difficult to take your kids to school and attend their many activities when you are a dialysis patient. It is difficult to travel when you are a hemodialysis patient because dialysis centers barely have enough machines and other resources for their own patients.

Terri Godwin was a city official in the District of Columbia when she realized that she could break this monotonous cycle that Natasha was living through in Durham, North Carolina. Knowing that Natasha would have to wait as many as seven years for her name to reach the top of the waiting list containing tens of thousands of patients waiting for kidneys from deceased donors, Terri proactively heeded the call and volunteered to donate one of her healthy kidneys to Natasha. *Natasha's Joy* details the love shared between sisters that made this miracle possible.

Living organ donors are special individuals. Although they come from all religions, races, genders, political parties, and socioeconomic classes, living donors share the unique gift of genuine altruism. There are no medical benefits, either physical or financial, for living donors who provide the lifesaving gifts of kidneys or parts of their livers. They willingly face the risk of death in an attempt to prolong the lives of their loved ones. Medical science cannot measure the psychological satisfaction they receive knowing that they gave the gift of life.

Bradley H. Collins, MD, FACS
Transplant Surgeon
Duke University Medical Center

Preface

$\mathcal{I}$ remember the day my sister Natasha was diagnosed with Lupus. Our lives were changed forever. Effects of the crippling disease caused achy joints, swelling, chronic fever, inflammation, high blood pressure, poor circulation, and skin rashes eventually resulting in kidney failure. There was no cure. Natasha, a second-grade teacher molding and shaping young minds, would be tied to a machine for the rest of her life if she did not receive a kidney transplant.

Natasha's diagnosis is not unique. All too often people everywhere are being controlled by machines or dying preventable deaths. Across the United States, there are about 97,000 candidates waiting for a life saving organ. Based on Organ Procurement and Transplantation Network (OPTN) data, at the time of this writing there are 27,000 African Americans waiting for a kidney.

Thankfully, for Natasha there is a brighter future. With the support of my family, the unwavering faith of our mother, and the unconditional love Natasha and I shared, a miracle happened.

If you are struggling with the decision to donate, if you are a dialysis patient considering transplantation, or a family member of a loved one awaiting a transplant, this book is written for you.

At the end of each chapter, the journal exercises will allow you to reflect and write about your thoughts and feelings as Natasha and I often did to help cope with our emotions.

It is my hope that this book will guide and inspire you. If you are capable of donating, I sincerely hope that you will become someone's miracle in the most meaningful life experience ever.

There is more life where my sister is.

—ANNE MORROW LINDBERGH

Chapter One

My Sister

Natasha is the oldest of us three girls born to Bettie Godwin, a praying mother, and Cary Godwin, a preaching father. Soon after Natasha arrived, Mom was pregnant with me. Just fifteen months apart, Natasha and I quickly bonded. We lived in Wilmington, North Carolina, the first few years so Dad could be close to his job. By the time Natasha was ready to start kindergarten we had moved to Ash, a small farming community fifty miles from Wilmington and twenty-five miles from Myrtle Beach, South Carolina. We had only one stoplight, a post office, and a handful of corner stores. Except for the time she went away to college, Mom had grown up and lived there most of her life. Mom's mother, Essie Bowens, lived across the road. Our great-grandma Ruth and Papa Roosevelt lived next door. From my earliest memories, other than my mother and father, they were the three adults on my mother's side who were a constant in my childhood. Dad's parents, my grandpa Charles and grandma Katie, lived about two hours away. We'd often go for visits, and Dad would bring them to spend summers with us. My Sioux Indian great-great-grandma Polly Marlow, Papa Roosevelt's mother, died a year before I was born. She had lived to be 106 years old. Mom spoke fondly of her infinite wisdom and wise counsel. Kin and neighbors, young and old, had flocked to her side daily for guidance.

We were blessed to share a close relationship with our grandparents. A narrow grassy path from the edge of our front yards connected the two brick homes. It was a path I walked many times, often to find Grandma Ruth sitting on the couch reading from a large-print Bible on her lap. Biblical literature, Bibles, and religious paintings adorned each room. God was recognized constantly, be it grace before a meal, a prayer of safety before a trip, or nightly bedtime appeals to the heavens above. Grandma Ruth didn't have a lot, but always managed to give presents or a small token gift to let us know she cared. She kept sweet potato pudding, rock candy, or fruit in the cupboard to offer when we came by. "Don't you young'uns want something to eat?" she would ask. She'd give the shirt off her back and her last dollar to whoever needed it. Papa Roosevelt and

Grandma Ruth were pillars of the small community and a refuge for many.

Mom met Dad on a visit to Philadelphia in the summer of 1965, and the two fell in love. Raised in a small town called Godwin, North Carolina, Dad was visiting his brother Charles and sister Mary who lived in

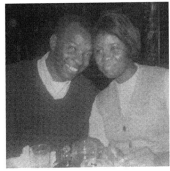

Mom and Dad in Mountain View, California, 1969.

Philadelphia. Then a student at North Carolina Agriculture and Technical State University, Dad had gone to Philadelphia to work and earn extra money to pay for school. He had been in school a year before being drafted into the Marines. Shortly after, Dad received orders to go to Vietnam. He and Mom courted mostly by mail while Dad was overseas. The two tied the knot on June 20, 1969. Then Mom moved with Dad to Mountain View, California, where he was stationed at Moffett Field Naval Air Station. To busy herself, she took a job as a bank teller. Mom often reminisced about the spectacular view of snow-covered mountains and neighboring valleys and how she wanted to take us on a cross-country trip there someday. After Dad's tour of duty they moved back to North Carolina. Mom stayed at home with us while Dad commuted to work each day at General

Electric in Wilmington. Growing up Natasha and I did everything together. We had fun doing things little girls do, from playing with dolls to drawing on mama's white walls. Mom loved to sew and made most of our clothes. She dressed us alike in frilly outfits with matching satin ribbons for our hair. Sewing and flower arranging were her two favorite hobbies. She'd spend hours in June's Fabric and Piece Goods picking out fabrics, matching up buttons, or browsing the many patterns in Butterick and Vogue. When word spread about Mom's craft, what was once a hobby quickly turned into full-time work. She'd stay up until the wee hours of the morning sewing a dress, pressing our hair, and ironing clothes. There are no words to express what an extraordinary, kind, and amazing woman she was. Her warm, friendly, and angelic nature instantly drew people to her. She was fun loving, generous, and entirely genuine. At five-foot-four with a caramel colored complexion and soft black hair, there was something very regal in the way she carried herself. Her style was simple yet elegant. She did so much for so many people in every aspect of her life. The time she took to prepare Sunday dinner, arrange a bouquet, or pick out a thank you card will not be forgotten. Her physical departure from this world on December 11, 2006, left us in shock and grief. However, for those of us who were blessed to know Mom, her spirit will live forever in our hearts and minds.

Mom taught us the value and power of prayer. And through her prayers Natasha and I have come to know the virtue of this divine art. Devout churchgoers, my parents took us to church every Sunday. Mom saw to it that we didn't miss a Sunday. Most of the time we sat quietly between Mom and Dad. When we were caught misbehaving, Mom would quietly lead us on tiptoe out of church, find the nearest bush, break off a twig, and make our legs dance. We marched back into church like little soldiers. By the time Mom joined the choir, we were old enough to sit quietly in the pews by ourselves.

Natasha was soft spoken, gentle, and kind—a lot like Mom. As my big sister she always looked out for me and I adored her. Everything she did, I thought I wanted to do until the summer we went away to camp. It was our first time away from home without Mom and Dad. Mom gathered our clothes and neatly packed the two little red suitcases she had bought us for the trip. By day three of the week-long girls camp, I was so homesick I didn't want to canoe; I didn't want to swim—I just wanted to go home. I cried and cried until the camp counselor let me call home. Natasha begged me to stay so we could get our camp certificate together, but

I just couldn't. Finally, Dad made the two-hour trek beyond the outskirts of Wilmington to pick me up. I packed my little red suitcase, said good-bye to Natasha, jumped in the car, and vowed never to go off to camp again!

In school Natasha learned to play the flute. I chose the clarinet. We took lessons in gymnastics, were taught piano, and stayed active in the 4-H Club. Mom persuaded Dad to buy us a piano so we could practice for our recitals at home. After dinner Natasha would excuse herself from the table, pull back the piano bench, and crank out the most beautiful rendition of "Swans on the Lake." It was her favorite. I leapt into a chair and gazed quietly as the classical tunes filled the room. The hooked-shaped musical notes required too much concentration for me. Natasha was disciplined and focused; I was mischievous and daring. Mom made sure we stayed active in programs that would stimulate our interests. *Little House on the Prairie* was our favorite TV show. Eight o'clock was our bedtime, but Mom would let us stay up an extra hour on Monday nights to watch the one-hour series.

When Natasha turned sixteen she got her license and Dad bought her a blue Chevy Chevette. She loved that little car. It had a stick shift, so the challenge was learning how to drive it. With a few lessons from Dad she was ready for the road. Dad let us drive to school each day. The next summer we got jobs at the Farmer's Daughter, a local seafood restaurant. Natasha drove us to work in the afternoons. The required dress was khaki pants and white polo shirts. The restaurant was fifteen minutes from where we lived in a nearby town called Calabash, North Carolina. Just minutes from Myrtle Beach, this small quaint wa-

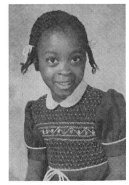

Natasha in Kindergarten.

terfront town hugs the South Carolina border. Touted as the "Seafood Capital of the World," Calabash is known for its vast array of seafood restaurants that line each avenue. There one can savor everything from fried fish and hush puppies cooked in a unique batter to clams and oysters on the half-shell all fresh off the docks. It was our favorite spot on Sunday afternoon.

When it came time for college, I didn't know where I wanted to go, let alone what I wanted to do. Natasha knew exactly what she wanted her career to be. She was always more driven than I was. She expressed early her desire to become a teacher and initially chose Campbell University to pursue her studies. The summer following graduation Mom drove Natasha to Buies Creek, North Carolina, to visit Campbell University where she intended to start in the fall. After the campus visit and orientation Natasha had a change of heart and decided she wanted to look elsewhere. Mom left Buies Creek and drove Natasha to Durham to visit North Carolina Central University. Mom had lived in Durham while attending Durham Business College. Knowing that the university had produced some of the nation's top African American professionals, Natasha immediately fell in love with the historically black college and its picturesque campus. When she thought about its strong liberal arts tradition, Natasha decided that North Carolina Central University would be her future, and she never looked back.

The next year I followed her. Natasha and I began our roller-coaster ride through college, rooming together on campus and later sharing an apartment. We learned how to cook our own meals, sort our own laundry, work, and keep up with schoolwork all at the same time. Mom and Dad made numerous trips up and down I-40 and Highway 55 to check on us. In between, Mom would write to us and Dad would send us money. "I love you. Don't forget to pray," they would always end their notes. We learned the joys of fighting over the most trivial things like whose turn it was to sweep the floor or wash the dishes. When we did fight, Natasha was always the first to apologize. Mom taught us never to be too proud to admit being wrong. And when I was wrong, Natasha was always quick to forgive. We learned so much about life together.

Shortly after graduation Natasha landed her first teaching job at Woodland Elementary in Roxboro. After two years at Woodland with an hour's commute each way, she began teaching second grade at Pearsontown Elementary School in Durham. During her tenure there she was in a car accident. She was riding with a college buddy in Myrtle Beach when the two were struck by a van. Natasha phoned Dad and a cousin who lived nearby. Dad rushed to South Carolina and drove them to the emergency room. They were released later that night. A few weeks after the accident, Natasha suddenly became ill. One evening while she was kneeling to meditate as she did at the end of each day, I noticed a ring of red spots around her right ankle. We drove to the emergency room. The doctor examined Natasha and at first suspected Lyme disease. He asked if we owned a pet or had been near any wooded areas. I thought about Shadow, my pet Sheltie, who often lounged in the living room.

The doctor performed a thorough examination that showed no visible signs of a tick bite. Natasha was treated with a series of antibodies and returned home. A few months later she began experiencing joint aches, occasional swelling in her hands, and fluid retention in her ankles. She developed chronic headaches. When she caught a cold, it took her weeks to recover. She had test after test and made countless trips to the ER. This treatment went on for several months before Natasha was referred to Dr. Nancy Allen, a rheumatologist who diagnosed the illness as an autoimmune disorder.

Dr. Allen began treating Natasha with prednisone, a steroid used to keep down inflammation. She prescribed blood pressure pills to control the hypertension and a special ointment for the patch of tiny red bumps that had surfaced on her forehead. This treatment kept the symptoms at bay, but something else was wrong.

Still puzzled and after weeks of more probing and another series of tests, Dr. Allen broke the devastating news. Natasha showed symptoms of lupus. I had heard of the illness but never really understood anything about it.

Lupus is an autoimmune disease that forces the body to attack its own cells and tissues, causing inflammation, joint pain, and, ultimately, organ damage. Statistics show the disease is more prevalent among people of color, including African Americans, Hispanics, Asians, and Native Americans, and develops most often in women. Medical experts maintain it is often difficult to recognize because symptoms mimic common diseases. Currently there is no cure. However, proper medical treatment can help keep the disease under control. According to the Lupus Foundation of America the treatments for symptoms may cause other health problems that in many patients can be worse than the disease itself.

Natasha taught for almost two years before the lupus began affecting her body internally. Fatigued and often in pain, she found it difficult to keep up with her daily routine. Along with the team of doctors who cared for Natasha, Mom remained our savior throughout this confusing and heartbreaking discovery. She dropped everything, packed her bags, and moved to Durham to care for Natasha. She enrolled our younger sister Katie in a nearby school. For more than a year she worked around the clock helping to care for Natasha until she was back on her feet. Dad stayed at home to work and drove up on weekends to visit.

After a kidney biopsy Natasha underwent chemotherapy in an attempt to stabilize her condition. Consecutive Plasmaphoresis treatments were performed, a process that can take up to several hours. The medical procedure involved exchanging Natasha's blood plasma (the watery part of blood) with a replacement solution. In this procedure, first blood is withdrawn so that the plasma can be separated from the blood cells. Once separated, the blood cells are recombined with a replacement solution that resembles plasma. The new mixture is then returned to the body through another tube. Doctors had to convince Natasha to stop working while she underwent treatment. At the end of six months her creatine level had improved enough to halt chemotherapy.

One Saturday morning in April 2001, we drove to Charlotte, North Carolina, for a wedding. Too tired to drive back after the long afternoon, we stayed the night there. Later that evening Natasha dropped off to sleep and woke up gasping for breath. I awoke, swung my legs off the bed, and hurried over to her side. We sat there for moment trying to figure out what was wrong. I grabbed whatever pillows I could find and propped them behind her head to see if that would temporarily relieve the discomfort. She settled back off to sleep, tossing and turning most of the night. Every time she moved, I jumped. On Sunday morning around 5 a.m., barely able to hold my eyes open, I propped a pillow behind my neck, put my head back, and finally drifted off to sleep. We slept a few hours and then checked out of the hotel, making the four-hour trip home to visit Mom and Dad. Katie was on Easter break. We stayed a couple of days and then drove back to Durham with Mom and young Katie in tow.

The next day we took Natasha to the emergency room. Her loss of kidney functions was causing excessive fluid build-up in her body and around her lungs making it difficult to breathe. After testing her creatine levels doctors made the grim discovery: Natasha was developing end stage renal disease. The lupus was attacking her kidneys. With barely any kidney functions, her body could become polluted with toxic materials. Doctors immediately started Natasha on dialysis. A surgeon inserted a catheter into her chest on the right just under the collarbone. Three days a week, nurses and technicians connected her to a ghastly-looking machine. It was ugly, but it kept her alive. They remained hopeful that her kidney functions might eventually be restored.

After a few months on dialysis her kidney functions had not improved. Natasha didn't like traveling much with her dialysis schedule, but she wanted to go home for Christmas as we did every year. The clinic social worker made some calls and located a dialysis center in nearby Myrtle Beach where she could receive treatment.

Dialysis was often painful to endure and to watch. It caused cramping, nausea, and often left Natasha weak and fatigued. On days she felt up to it, she would drive herself to the clinic. It gave her a sense of independence. Still, I couldn't help but feel sad and completely helpless as I watched her hopes, dreams, and ambitions slowly fade. Treatment after treatment she never complained. Her spirit was strong, yet I sensed her suffering.

Dr. Steven Smith at Duke Hospital made the suggestion that Natasha consider transplantation. She had two options: remain on dialysis for the rest of her life or get a kidney transplant that could quite possibly return her life to normal. He arranged for us to meet Leslie Hicks, a transplant coordinator. During the meeting Leslie discussed the steps involved in becoming a candidate for kidney transplantation. The average wait on the National Donor List was three to seven years. Leslie suggested that a family member consider donating. Dad and Mom immediately volunteered, but because of their health history they were not qualified. Our cousin Angela, Natasha's best friend, offered to be a backup.

Petrified at the thought of donating a kidney and what the future implications might be, still there was no question in my mind. I had to help Natasha survive—for my family, the many children whose lives she had yet to touch, and me. Frightened by the potentially risky procedure, Natasha quickly rejected the idea. Neither she nor I had had any children, and I wondered if having only one kidney would lessen my chance of becoming a mother. I prayed and prayed to God, researched living donation, and sought counsel from family and friends. Natasha needed my kidney, and if she didn't get it she would be tied to a machine for the rest of her life.

It was becoming increasingly clear. Donation was the only thing left to do. I went on planning. Meanwhile, Natasha continued her prayers for total divine healing, hoping an operation wouldn't be necessary. Then it finally sank in. God wanted to heal Natasha, but he wanted to use my kidney to perform the miracle.

Not quite convinced surgery was the answer, one bright Sunday morning, feeling achy and tired, Natasha got dressed for church. She arrived a few minutes late for the 8:00 a.m. service and was ushered to the front row. Dr. Fletcher, who was ministering, stopped halfway through his teaching and pointed to Natasha in the crowded sanctuary. "Natasha," he said, "God is going to perform that miracle in your body. When God gives you this brand new kidney you will be completely off dialysis. Don't be afraid, God has already finished it." Natasha rose slowly to her feet, clapping in a small flutter of excitement. Having struggled with the thoughts of a transplant, she finally felt at peace.

Meditation

"I can do all things through Christ who strengthens me."

—PHILIPPIANS 4:13

This was one of Natasha's favorite meditations as she was going through the many challenges of her illness. She would often say this to herself, and it became a part of her healing process no matter how bleak her prognosis looked.

Activity

Take some time to write down your favorite mediations in the space below and refer to them whenever you need the strength to stay positive and keep going.

_____

_____

_____

_____

_____

_____

_____

_____

_____

_____

_____

_____

_____

_____

_____

_____

_____

_____

_____

_____

_____

_____

_____

_____

_____

_____

_____

_____

_____

_____

_____

Chapter Two

Becoming a Match

The first step in the transplant process was to determine if our blood types matched. Leslie scheduled a litany of tests for Natasha and me, involving blood typing, tissue sampling, and cross matching. I had jitters when she finally phoned with the results. If I were a match, could I really go through with it? If I were not a match, where would we turn? What would happen to Natasha's quality of life if she had to endure years of waiting to reach the top of the national donor's list? All of these thoughts swirled in my head.

Finally the results were in and the tests were positive. Three out of six of our antigens matched. This was great news. It meant that Natasha would have a much greater chance of accepting the kidney at the time of donation. The marathon began with intense all-day work-ups, physical exams, x-rays, more blood tests, and interviews with a social worker. Topics covered everything from risks involved to finances and family support. They offered me a way to back out if I changed my mind, but I assured them I was prepared to go through with it. No guarantees were made but every precaution was taken by the transplant team to ensure that I understood the total scope and long-term implications of what could occur. Risks from the surgery itself can include blood-clotting, hemorrhaging, infections, injury to other organs, and, in rare cases, death. Health professionals maintain that donating a kidney generally does not increase the risks of future health problems or decrease life expectancy. However, living donors should be aware that if something happens to the one remaining kidney, such as a severe trauma, kidney function could be compromised. Special measures should be taken, such as proper diet, monitoring of sodium intake to avoid hypertension, and keeping the remaining kidney healthy.

According to the *Wall Street Journal* living donation has risen in recent years. So has growing concern that donors themselves face significant medical, psychological, and financial risk. Laura Meckler's article in the *Wall Street Journal* reported that more than 7,000 people became living donors in 2005, triple the number just a decade ago. Patient advocates argue that hospitals and federal agencies aren't doing enough to inform living donors of the consequences of such noble acts. The first successful living donor transplant was performed in 1954, and has proven safe for most donors, though some do later suffer from medical setbacks. The *Wall Street Journal* article reported that out of more than 50,000 live kidney transplants from 1987 to 2002, fifty-six (56) kidney donors in the U.S. are known to have later needed transplants themselves.

Requirements for transplantation candidacy also stipulated that Natasha raise money to finance the first year of anti-rejection drugs required after transplants. Known as immunosuppressants, anti-rejection drugs are costly and work to prevent the body from rejecting the new kidney. Rejection occurs when the body recognizes that the transplanted kidney is not its own and mobilizes the immune system to fight against it. Studies show that rejection is more common in the early months, but can occur at anytime.

According to an article in the *Congressional Quarterly*, healthcare professionals say hospitals occasionally do refuse to perform transplants or add people to organ waiting lists if they can't demonstrate an ability to pay for the transplant surgery, which can cost as much as $300,000.

Together with a few friends we established a kidney fund. Natasha loved to read so I created bookmarks and mailed them to close friends and family. We raised just over

$1,000, enough to get us started. Then Dr. Bradley Collins told Natasha about a clinical trial being conducted on some of the immunosuppressant therapies she would require. It would allow her to receive the medicines she needed without the cost until clinical research on the treatment was complete. He suggested she participate, and Natasha quickly agreed.

In early March, I met Dr. Kuo, the surgeon who would perform my procedure. He reviewed my chart and discussed the laparoscopic procedure, which would involve an incision below the belly button and three smaller incisions up to half an inch on the left side. Plastic tubes called ports are pushed through these incisions. A camera is used to monitor the procedure, and surgical instruments are threaded through the ports, used to remove the kidney and tie off the blood vessels. The old technique required surgeons to make a six- to ten-inch cut in the patient's side, maneuver through three muscle layers, and cut out part of the ribs to get to the kidney.

To ensure I was physically fit for the challenge, Dr. Kuo suggested I get to work on shedding a few pounds. I was much plumper than Natasha, and the less fat there is in the stomach area, the quicker things tend to heal and the less invasive the surgery. After the advice about losing weight Dr. Kuo encouraged me to stay active and resume a light exercise routine after the surgery, as soon as I felt up to it. This would improve my strength and endurance while providing the necessary therapy to get me back on my feet. He described me as "an athlete in training." Since crash diets had never worked for me, on the days I came home early enough I strolled around a nearby track.

Natasha had always maintained a neat figure. After being diagnosed with lupus she was put on prednisone to control the inflammation. She'd occasionally gain a pound or two depending on the dosage prescribed. When her kidney functions started deteriorating Natasha began retaining fluid in her tummy area. At one point she looked to be five months pregnant. She was so uncomfortable that one night Mom and I rushed her to the ER. Doctors made a small incision and drained several quarts of fluid from her belly. The next day Dr. Allen was furious and maintained it would only reaccumulate. Fortunately it didn't. By the time we were ready for surgery Natasha had dropped to a size four. The weight loss was attributed to diet restrictions associated with the dialysis treatment.

With under two months before surgery, fear and anger was taking its toll on me. I had never been a hospital patient for any reason, let alone surgery. The slightest prick of a needle sent me into a frenzy. What will happen to me afterwards? Natasha's body could reject my kidney. What if something happened during the surgery? Will I die? Could I stand that much pain? What will my stomach look like afterwards? How ugly will the scars be? This was scary stuff! The more I thought about it the more scared I became. Despite all the fuss about my bravery, I was far from it.

As we neared the date for surgery, more tests were performed. I was living in Washington, DC, and commuted back and forth to North Carolina for testing. In April 2002, I flew back to Durham for the angiogram, the only test that was slightly painful. My parents drove up to be with me for the procedure.

The angiogram involved an injection of dye into the artery. It sends a warm feeling through the body—like a hot flash. With the computer screen next to me, I could literally see my kidneys. The angiogram helps the surgeon determine which kidney to remove. After climbing down from the table, I started to itch. Light pink patches popped up on my legs. It was hives. My body was allergic to the intravenous dye used to enhance the image of my kidney on x-ray film. Ordered by the nurse, I downed two doses of Benedryl and in a few minutes the hives started to fade. Results of the angiogram showed that my kidneys were in good condition. To avoid another trip to Durham, Leslie scheduled my final work-up to be performed at Howard University Transplant Center. The results were then sent back to Duke. The transplant was on schedule for June 12, a few days shy of Mom's 55th birthday.

Fear and Anger

$\mathcal{I}$t is normal to be afraid of giving away part of your body. When the fear and anger started taking a toll on me, I would not only pray and meditate, but also talk with close family members, friends, and even other donors and recipients. I sought counsel from our pastor and surrounded myself with positive people.

Activity

Think about a time when fear and anger took hold of you, for whatever reason. What did you do to stay calm? Write it down.

_____

_____

_____

_____

_____

_____

_____

_____

Chapter Three

Financial Barriers

Lost wages and time off from work are the most noted barriers living donors face when deciding to donate. The recipient's health coverage generally pays for the donor's medical costs such as surgery and pre- and post-op tests. But donors themselves are responsible for their own, if any, travel expenses, trips to the hospital, hotel rooms, follow-up care, wages lost while they recuperate, and any medical problems down the road.

According to an article in the *Washington Post* dated March 20, 2007, transplant advocates fear that costs to the donor are a deterrent to donating, and continue searching for ways to compensate living donors who can donate kidney, bone marrow, or other organs. Advocates see donor tax breaks as the government's responsibility and continue to lobby Congress for greater incentives.

The National Conference of State Legislatures maintains that eleven states, beginning with Wisconsin, have passed laws providing a $10,000 tax deduction for living donors to help cover uncompensated expenses. The following states in the chart below have passed legislation related to living organ donation.

State Tax Deductions and Donor Leave Laws

State	Law	Comments
Arkansas	$10,000 Organ Donation Tax Deduction*	Signed into law on March 9, 2005.
Georgia	$10,000 Organ Donation Tax Deduction*	Signed into law on April 29, 2004.
Hawaii	Leave of absence for organ and bone marrow donors	
Idaho	State employee leave of absence and income tax credit for live organ donation expenses	Signed into law on July 1, 2006.
Iowa	$10,000 Organ Donation Tax Deduction*	Signed into law on May 12, 2005.
Minnesota	$10,000 Organ Donation Tax Deduction*	Signed into law on July 14, 2005.
Mississippi	$10,000 Organ Donation Tax Deduction*	
Missouri	Paid Leave of Absence	State employees are allowed paid leave for living organ donors (30 days) and marrow donors (5 days).
New Mexico	$10,000 Organ Donation Tax Deduction*	Signed into law on April 5, 2005.
New York	$10,000 Organ Donation Tax Deduction*	Signed into law on August 16, 2006.

North Dakota	$10,000 Organ Donation Tax Deduction*	Signed into law on March 14, 2005.
Ohio	Liver, kidney, or bone marrow donor leave and $10,000 Organ Donation Tax Deduction*	
Oklahoma	Organ Donor Education and Awareness Program (ODEAP) and $10,000 Organ Donation Tax Deduction*	
Texas	Paid Leave of Absence	HB89 bill allows state employees up to 30 days paid leave to donate an organ, five days for bone marrow donation, and up to one hour per quarter to donate blood (with their supervisor's permission).
Utah	$10,000 Organ Donation Tax Deduction*	Signed into law on March 21, 2005.
Virginia	Paid Leave of Absence	State employees are allowed up to thirty days of paid leave in any calendar year, in addition to other paid leave, to serve as bone marrow or organ donors.
Wisconsin	$10,000 Organ Donation Tax Deduction and Paid Leave of Absence	

*Law allows living organ donors to deduct as much as $10,000 on their state income taxes for travel, lodging, and lost wages related to the donation. The law applies to donations of a liver, pancreas, kidney, intestine, or bone marrow from living donors only.

Source: http://www.transplantliving.org

This chart was originally created on March 14, 2005, by the United Network for Organ Sharing and last modified on December 11, 2007.

At the time of my donation I had been working in city government sixteen months before discovering I did not have enough leave accrued to take the six weeks needed to recover. I exhausted what leave I had left and prepared to put myself on a tight budget for the period I would be without pay. Colleagues who learned of my plight joined forces and donated seventy-eight hours of their own paid vacation time so that I would continue receiving a salary while recovering from surgery. I was totally moved by the kind gesture. The *Washington Post* published a story about the city workers in the August 15, 2002, issue of the *Washington Post District Weekly.*

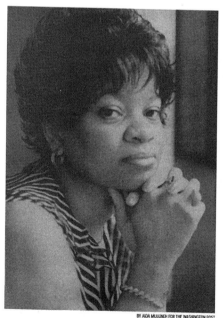

BY AIDA MULUNEH FOR THE WASHINGTON POST

Terri Godwin, an aide to the mayor, donated a kidney to her sister.

The Washington Post

DISTRICT
EXTRA

THURSDAY, AUGUST 15, 2002

Helping a Helper

D.C. Workers Give Vacation Time To Colleague Who Donated Kidney

By C. EDWARD WALKER
Special to The Washington Post

When Mayor Anthony A. Williams's chief Web master decided to donate a kidney to her ailing sister in North Carolina, her District colleagues got together and gave her what employees nationwide might consider their most precious asset: time off.

"It's not just, can we get by without her for a couple of months?" said communications director Tony Bullock. "There was a desire to help her financially."

Four of the six members of the mayor's communications staff donated 78 hours of paid vacation to make sure that Terri Godwin would receive her salary while she recovered from surgery to donate a kidney to her sister, Natasha.

The vacation hours were not just lost to travel or to relaxation. The city allows employees to convert unused vacation time into cash.

"It was just no way I couldn't do it," said senior speechwriter Betsy

SISTERS Page 6

49

City Workers Pitch In for Colleague Who Donated Kidney

SISTERS, *From Page 3*

Peoples, who at the time was planning a wedding and a honeymoon. "I just thought [giving her kidney] was the most unselfish act that anyone could do. I was speechless."

Her colleagues' gestures left Godwin deeply moved. "I was just humbled," she said.

This story of love and sacrifice has it roots in North Carolina where Terri, 30, and Natasha, 32, were reared in a close-knit religious family. They studied and roomed together at North Carolina Central University and shared an apartment until Terri took up Web operations in the District in 2001.

Earlier this month, still sore after the operation, Terri was beaming at her sister's newfound joy and health. She shared post-surgery pictures: Natasha smiling and a somber Terri holding a pillow over her incisions.

The doctors had told the sisters that Natasha would be more energized by the transplant because her body had hit a low and Terri would be more pained because her body had been healthy. But sacrifice trumps pain, Terri said.

"To give your sister life is one of the greatest gifts you can give," she said. "It makes me feel good to see her being up and having more energy."

In the long term, health officials say, there is a chance that the donated kidney could fail. But for today, Natasha Godwin feels "wonderful . . . just like I've been reborn," she said in a recent interview from her home in Durham, N.C.

In 1997, Natasha, a former second-grade teacher, first noticed symptoms of lupus, an autoimmune disease. She had gone to seek treatment for minor injures suffered in an auto accident. But by the time the episode ended, she could not return to work.

As the disease became worse, Natasha was sometimes unable to walk or breathe. But the Godwin family supported her throughout the ordeal, nursing her and helping out with money.

Natasha said she prayed but at times felt like conceding defeat.

Last year, Terri decided to donate a kidney. But as the June 12 transplant date neared, she said, she had plenty of last-minute jitters.

"I was petrified," she said. "I was so scared."

Colleagues helped her through the ordeal.

"I told her that God was smiling at her," Peoples said. "No one would be able to do something as loving as this without Him."

Lateef Mangum, audio/visual specialist and photographer for the mayor's office, put in a special plea to his sister, who works at Duke University Medical Center in Durham, where the transplant was performed, to make sure that the sisters received the best care.

"I don't really even consider what I did of major significance," Mangum said. "The real hero is Terri Godwin."

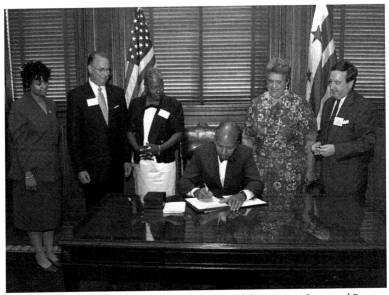

On August 5, 2002, Mayor Anthony Williams signed the District's Organ and Bone Marrow Donor Leave Amendment Act. The bill grants city employees up to 30 days paid leave when they serve as a living organ or bone marrow donor.

(Left to right) Terri Godwin, Ronald Paul, former Ward 8 Councilmember Sandy Allen, former DC Mayor Anthony Williams, Virginia Williams, Preston Englert, Jr. President/ CEO NFK of the National Capital Area.

On August 5, 2002, two months after my surgery, my boss, Mayor Anthony Williams, formerly signed into law the Organ Donor Leave Act, granting city employees thirty days paid leave when they serve as organ or bone marrow donors. I had recently returned to work when asked to join Mayor Williams and the city councilmembers for the bill signing ceremony. I was honored just to be in the room. But when asked to speak, I thanked Mayor Williams and the city council for their support of the bill, my colleagues who had joined me for the ceremony, and all those involved in the effort.

When living donors don't have to worry about bills getting paid, that's one less hurdle to cross. The district joined states nationwide replicating the federal legislation passed in 1999. In April 2006, DC Council member Carol Schwartz introduced a similar bill. The proposed legislation would establish a credit for corporate taxpayers and businesses who allow an employee up to thirty days paid leave to serve as a living organ donor and up to seven days paid leave to serve as a bone marrow donor without loss or reduction in pay, earned vacation leave, or credit for time of service. The legislation became effective March 6, 2007.

Journal Your Thoughts

As Natasha prayed and meditated, she also kept a journal and wrote about her feelings, pain, and anything else that came up. Below are some of Natasha's reflections.

When I had my prayer and quiet time, I wrote about what I was feeling, emotionally and physically. I often listened to praise and worship music during this time. After prayer and worship time, I jotted down what the Lord had spoken to me as I communicated with him. Afterwards I always felt better emotionally and mentally, even if I didn't feel physically better. I wrote a lot during my illness.

Activity

In the space provided, write down any feelings as they come up and don't hesitate to share them with others. You can also encourage family members, friends, and your medical team to jot down their feelings and wishes for you on the following pages.

_____

_____

_____

Chapter Four

The Transplant

After only a few hours of sleep, early on Tuesday, June 11, 2002, I packed the car and headed for North Carolina, arriving in time for my pre-operative work-up. I thought to myself if only I had listened to Mom who had urged me to come a few days early to rest up before the big day. I was a basket case when I left the pre-op station. Luvae Wall, the nurse now in charge of my screening, became worried. She volunteered to stop by after her shift to check on me. After the screening, my mom and I drove back to my sister's place where I would take the rest of the day to relax. Luvae stopped by just as she had promised. Surprised by her visit, we gathered in the living room, chatted, and quietly listened as she tried to soothe our fears. Later that evening a few of Natasha's church friends stopped by and had prayer with us.

I awoke at 6:00 a.m. cranky, tired, and scared. I was getting dressed when Natasha turned to me and said, "If you don't want to go through with it, I'll understand." I was petrified, but couldn't bear the thought of Natasha enduring another day of dialysis. Mom was busy getting dressed and dialing her prayer partners.

Dad drove us to the hospital. Mom and I went back to the dressing room first. The nurse handed me a gown and cap and told Mom to wait in the lounge area. Tears flooded my eyes and my voice choked as I looked up at the nurse. Mom took my hand and whispered a prayer. Then the nurse turned to Mom and said she could go on back with me. I changed out of my clothes into the hospital gown. Mom bundled my braids into the cap the nurse had given me. "I wish I had some scissors to cut these things off so your neck doesn't get a cramp," she said. My surgery was first. Natasha stayed with me until it was her turn to go back. We sat quietly in the waiting room. Natasha held my hand and prayed that I would be okay. She thanked me for being so brave.

Everyone hovered around to wish me well. Minutes before the nurse wheeled me back to the operating room, my college mentor, Dr. Beverly Jones, breezed through the door, smiling. We hugged and exchanged pleasantries.

Then she wished me well. The anesthesiologist checked me over one last time. I waved goodbye as they ushered me down the hall. The transplant was becoming a reality. In a few hours Natasha would have a healthy kidney. Doctors warned that the kidney could reject, or may not start to work right away. Excited and nervous I tried not to think about it. The anesthesiologist looked down at me, smiled, and gently rubbed my hand. I whispered one last prayer and felt a peace and a confidence that everything was now in God's hands.

Three hours later I awoke in the recovery room, shivering in a warm blanket. What had hit me? I wondered. I was groggy and in intense pain. The folly catheter that had been inserted to drain my bladder was so uncomfortable it hurt to move. My surgery lasted about three hours and Natasha's surgery lasted close to five hours. The surgical team later explained that Natasha's surgery had run longer to compensate for the extra artery on my kidney discovered during surgery. This meant that Natasha's surgeon, Dr. Collins, had to take the extra time to connect in the additional artery from my kidney.

I was taken from the recovery room up to another floor and into a regular hospital room. My eyes opened slowly as faint voices entered the room. I looked up, pushed the pain control pump, and continued to drift in and out of consciousness. With his team, Dr. Kuo came over and stood next to my bedside. He pulled back the covers and looked me over. I was anxious to hear how Natasha was. She was in the intensive care unit with Mom and Dad standing next to her bedside. She gripped both their hands and felt them squeeze hers. In a soft whisper, Natasha said, "I love you Mom and Dad, thank you for all you have done for me."

Dr. Kuo said the transplant was successful. The kidney went right to work, making urine on the operating table. It was a miracle! A sigh of relief came over me. Then everything in the room grew quiet as he explained that during the operation my spleen was accidentally nicked. My head spontaneously snapped up and my heart sank. Dr. Kuo assured me I would be okay. The nick had been repaired with fibrin glue and he was confident it would gradually mend

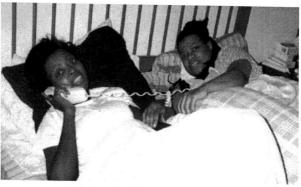

Natasha and Terri recovering at home.

itself. That evening Mom and Dad wheeled me down to see Natasha. She was in pain, but each day she seemed to get stronger. She received flowers, notes, and many well wishes. I went home on Friday, two days after the surgery. Natasha was doing so well that she was released on Saturday, days earlier than the doctors had expected.

Mom worked overtime cooking, cleaning, making prescription runs, and nursing us back to health. By the end of the next week Natasha was up making breakfast and walking around. I had to stay in bed a good deal of the time and couldn't understand why my body was in such a slump.

When I went back for my follow up, Dr. Kuo explained that living donors typically experience a longer and harder recuperation period. Natasha was more energized because prior to her surgery her body

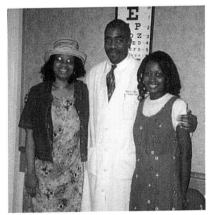

A few weeks after surgery.
(Left to right) Terri Godwin, Dr. Bradley Collins, and Natasha Godwin.

had hit a low. I was more in pain because my body had been healthy and was suddenly traumatized.

When we were growing up, family gatherings were routine. A week after our surgery two carloads of my relatives, including great-aunt Rudell, drove up to stay the weekend with us. They gave Mom a much-needed break. As they sat around laughing, talking, and reminiscing about old times, the aroma of fresh greens and stewed chicken filled the air. Everyone was happy to see us recuperating well.

Intangible Benefits

I consider myself extremely fortunate to have been able to help Natasha by donating a kidney to her. Knowing that I helped her resume a normal life and get back to doing the things she loved doing without being tied to a machine brings my heart great joy. I also benefited by knowing I did the right thing spiritually. I answered God's call. *At the end of each day when I see my sister smile, I feel I have received a far greater gift than I gave.*

Activity

If you are a donor, make a list of the positive benefits you feel at having enabled someone to enjoy the quality of life that many take for granted.

_____

_____

_____

_____

_____

_____

Natasha's Joy

Chapter Five

Life after Donation

*I*t's been five years since my kidney donation. In December, seven months after the surgery, Dr. Collins removed an itchy keloid that had formed near my incision site. Keloids are thick, itchy clusters of scar tissue that develop from injury to the skin. Medical experts maintain that people who donate a kidney can live a normal life. Experts tell us that the remaining kidney increases in size to compensate for the loss of the donated kidney. Aside from the nagging ache on my left side, which comes and goes mostly when I over-exert myself or lift heavy objects, I have not experienced any complications. I get regular check-ups to monitor my kidney functions, drink plenty of water to prevent dehydration, watch my sodium intake, and steer clear of flag football. Natasha takes anti-rejection medicines daily and gets check-ups more regularly.

To mark our third year anniversary, on June 11, 2005, Mom, who was recovering from a surgery in May, hosted a celebration of thanksgiving. We tried to talk her out of it, but she wanted in her own special way to thank God and countless others who had helped us along the way. We named it our "kidneyversary." Mom loved gospel music so she lined up singers, invited church choirs, family, neighbors, ministers, and friends. Gathered under a giant white tent that covered the lawn of a park dedicated to my great-grandparents, we feasted on a delicious buffet of food and hummed to the soulful sounds of gospel. Chatter filled the air as everyone moved about shaking hands, hugging, and exchanging pleasantries. Standing at the podium with tears welling in her eyes, Mrs. Judy Evans, our English teacher in grade school, reminisced about how she came to know us. "I feel so blessed to know these girls and to be a part of this celebration," she said. Mrs. Evans was one of those teachers that would always bring a ray of sunshine into the classroom. She was warm, loving, friendly, and always made time for her students. Dusk began to fall. Soon after the guests declared they couldn't eat anymore, we finished up the celebration and returned home.

In the fall following her surgery, Natasha enrolled in graduate school at North Carolina Central University.

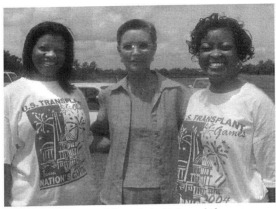

Natasha and Terri celebrate their third year kidneyversary.
(Left to right) Terri, Mrs. Judy Evans, and Natasha.

Two years later she graduated Summa Cum Laude, earning a master's degree in school administration. Natasha is passionate about teaching, learning, and helping children. Now she joyfully works as dean of students at the Josephine Dobbs-Clement Early College High School in North Carolina. She nicknamed the kidney "Joy" in honor of how appreciative she is for the new joy in her life. My family frequently jokes that Natasha has taken on many of my likes and dislikes. She thanks me often with trinkets, cards, and special handwritten notes. At the end of the day when I see Natasha smile, I know I have received a far greater gift than I gave.

Challenges and Triumphs

Of the many challenges I faced during the process of kidney donation, the most difficult was watching Natasha suffer with her illness. But there have been many triumphant moments since my donation. Among them was watching Natasha walk across the stage to receive her master's degree in school administration, a longtime dream of hers. In June 2007, we reached our five-year Kidneyversary, and Lord knows I am extremely grateful to have finished writing this book!

Activity

Can you recall a time when you faced a really tough situation? What about an achievement you are especially proud of? Write down some of the challenging and triumphant moments in your life, either before or after donation.

_____

_____

_____

_____

_____

Chapter Six

Why We Don't Donate

According to U.S. Census data, there are 38,342,549 African Americans in the United States. Based on The Organ Procurement and Transplantation Network Data, 27,000 African Americans remain on the national transplant waiting list. Despite continuing efforts at public education, misconceptions and inaccuracies about living donation still persist. African Americans are believed to be more reluctant to become donors often because of religious beliefs, misconception, fear, and lack of information.

A study conducted by Wake Forest University Medical Center reports that obesity and failure to complete the donor evaluation are the primary reasons blacks are less likely to become living donors. As part of the survey, 541 donor questions and charts for disqualified potential donors were reviewed. Findings revealed that 30 percent of blacks were excluded because of obesity, compared to 16.6 percent of whites.

When you're faced with a tough decision such as this, know the facts, follow your heart, and above all pray. When I see Natasha I'm reminded of my purpose on earth.

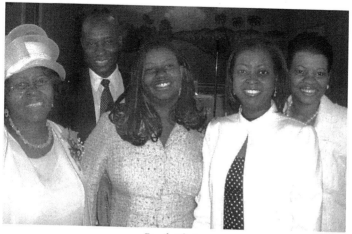

Family Photo.
(Left to right) Mom, Dad, Katie, Natasha, and Terri.

Count Your Blessings

According to Dr. Andrew Weil, keeping a "daily" gratitude journal for just two to three weeks has been shown to improve mental health and well-being in organ-transplant recipients.

Activity

If you are a recipient, take a few minutes each day to write down what you are thankful for. It could be some kind words you received from another or something you did that made you laugh or brought you joy.

_____

_____

_____

_____

_____

_____

_____

_____

Frequently Asked Questions

When was the first successful living donor transplant performed?

Dr. Joseph E. Murray performed the first successful living donor transplant in 1954. The transplant was performed on twenty-three-year-old identical twins.

Can a person live with one kidney?

Most people are born with two kidneys, and some are born with a single kidney. The kidneys act as the functional components of the renal system. They regulate blood pressure, produce red blood cells, activate vitamin D, and produce glucose. Experts maintain that we are born with an overabundance of kidney functions. If only one kidney is present, the remaining kidney will adjust to filter as much as two kidneys would normally. A single kidney with only 75 percent of its functional capacity can sustain life provided one maintains the proper diet and exercise. Evidence suggests that living kidney donors are highly unlikely to develop significant long-term detrimental effects to their health, as illustrated by donors whose renal function has been assessed for up to thirty years following donation. The main problems with donors are rare instances of complications having to do with the surgery, not lack of the kidney.

*W*hat are the advantages of a *living* donor kidney transplant?

Medical experts maintain that the chances of a successful transplant are better with living donor organs than those from deceased donors. It also eliminates the three- to five-year wait for a deceased-donor organ and longer time spent on hemodialysis.

*W*hat are the qualifications to be a living donor?

Living donor candidates should generally be between the ages of eighteen and sixty years old. Donors must be healthy, close to their ideal body weight, and not have high blood pressure, diabetes, or other significant health problems.

*W*hat are some of the risks associated with the donor's operation?

Risk from the surgery itself can include blood clotting, hemorrhaging, infection, injury to other organs, and, in rare cases, death.

*W*hat kind of follow-up care is important for living donors?

You should maintain regular check-ups with your family doctor to monitor your kidney functions. Proper diet and exercise are also important in keeping your kidney healthy.

*D*oes donating a kidney prevent you from becoming pregnant or fathering a child?

I have found no medical evidence in my research to suggest that donating a kidney has any effect on the ability of donors to have children. Doctors advise transplant recipients to wait six to twelve months before becoming pregnant.

*I*s it normal to be afraid of becoming a living donor?

Sure. It's very normal to experience feelings of fear about giving away a part of your body and to experience guilt about not wanting to donate.

My Questions

Additional Support Information and Resources for Living Donors

❧

*M*any organizations offer support and resources for potential living donors and recipients. The following list provides a guide to a wide range of these organizations, the services they offer as well as laws and legislation governing organ donation.

Washington Regional Transplant Community
http://www.wrtc.org
(866) 232-3666

United Network Organ Sharing
http://www.unos.com
(800) 355-Share

Minority Organ Tissue Transplant Education Program
(Mottep)
http://www.nationalmottep.org
(800) 393-2839

National Kidney Foundation
http://www.nkf.org
(800) 622-9010

Carolina Donor Services
www.carolinadonorservices.org
1-800-200-2672

The Organ Procurement and Transplant Network
www.optn.org

Transweb
www.transweb.org

OrganDonor.Gov
www.OrganDonor.gov

Donate Life America
www.donatelife.net

Selected Bibliography

Brody, Jane E. "For Living Donors, Many Risks to Weigh," *New York Times*, September 4, 2007.

Brody, Jane E. "The Solvable Problem of Organ Shortages," *New York Times*, August 28, 2007.

Feifer, Jason. "Paying Big to Be a Donor," *Washington Post,* March 20, 2007, HE01.

Hansen, Brian. "Organ Shortage," *The Congressional Quarterly Researcher*, 2003: Volume 13, No. 7, 153-76.

Meckler, Laura. "What Living Donors Need to Know," *Wall Street Journal*: January 30, 2007, B11.

Organ and Bone Marrow Donor Act of 2006, (March 6, 2007) sec. 47-1807.08.

"Population Estimates," DC Office of Planning http:// planning.dc.gov/. *Study Evaluates Why Blacks Do Not Successfully Donate Kidneys*," Wake Forest University Baptist, Medical Center, May 17, 2007. Http://www1. wfubmc.edu/News/NewsARticle.htm?ArticleID=2077

Title XII of the District of Columbia Comprehensive Merit Personnel Act of 1978, (December 3, 1979). DC Law 2-139; DC Official Code 1-612.01 *et. Seq. Organ and Bone Marrow Donor Leave Amendment Act of 2002,* sec. 1203b. Donor Leave, (2002).

Acknowledgments

I want to thank my loving parents, Cary and Bettie J. Godwin. Dad, your constant support, wisdom, and guidance helped me become the person I am today. Mom, your greatest gift to me was your unwavering faith in God. Without your constant support, nurturing, and prayer, I would not have achieved the successes I have. You are the true driving force in my life and it is because of you and your quest to help others I envisioned and wrote this book.

Special thanks to my editor, Gail Kearns of To Press and Beyond, for her expert insights, meticulous editing, and thoughtful creativity that has guided this book.

Thanks also to my former teacher Arthrell D. Sanders for her editorial contribution to this book.

To my sister Natasha, thank you for your constant encouragement, your positive spirit, and your Godly wisdom.

To my sister Katie, thank you for motivating me. I am so proud of the young lady you are becoming.

To my dear friend Betsy Adeboyejo, thank you for your friendship and inspired support throughout this project.

To all my family and friends too numerous to name, thank you for your love, support, and prayers.

To almighty God, thank you! thank you! thank you!

Reflections

For donors and recipients: As you look back on your journey, are there things you wish you had done differently? Are there things you are glad you did? Is there someone special you'd like to write about? Natasha, for example, wishes she had started walking and exercising a little more after the surgery.

I wish I had begun a steady workout regime six months before my donation. Looking back, I wish I had not been so consumed with fear and donated my kidney as soon as doctors determined Natasha needed a transplant.

Activity

This is the space in which to write some of your reflections and to give thanks to the people who helped you through your journey!

About the Author

$\mathcal{A}$ native of North Carolina, Terri Godwin is an advocate for living donation. A volunteer member of the Washington Regional Transplant Community, Terri has been involved with various initiatives to raise awareness and educate others about living donation. She testified before the Council of the District of Columbia in support of legislation to establish a tax credit for corporate taxpayers and businesses in the District of Columbia who allow employees time off without loss or reduction in pay when they serve as a bone marrow or living organ donor. The legislation became effective March 6, 2007.

Terri matriculated at North Carolina Central University earning a B.A. in History and M.A. in Educational Technology. In 2001, Terri moved to Washington, DC, where she served six years for DC Mayor Anthony Williams. She has worked as a communications officer, speech writer, and media spokesperson. Currently, Terri resides in North Carolina.